NAVIGATING SEXUAL WELLNESS

A COMPREHENSIVE GUIDE TO HOLISTIC SEXUAL HEALTH

AHMED .R

Contents

CHAPTER ONE 3

INTRODUCTION 3

The Basics of Sexual Health..5

The Evolution of Sexual Norms and Beliefs in Ancient
Civilizations 9

Europe in the Middle Ages: Sexuality, Sin, and Redemption 12

Revisiting the Body and the Self throughout the Renaissance
and Enlightenment...16

CHAPTER TWO 19

Victorian Ethics and the Development of Sexuality 20

Physiology and Anatomy of the Biological Basis of Sex 21

The Physiology of the Sexual Reaction....................................24

Resolve, orgasm, plateau, and excitement 24

Gender Identity and Sexual Orientation 27

Encouraging the Health of Sexuality 32

Taking Care of Sexual Disorders and Dysfunction....................38

Sexual dysfunction and disorders: categories..........................39

CHAPTER THREE 43

Increasing Satisfaction and Sexual Pleasure 45

Honest Communication 47

Investigating Sensuality 49

Healthy Sexual Behavior Throughout Life 51

Social and Cultural Aspects of Sexual Health 58

CHAPTER FOUR 67

Accepting Liberation and Authenticity in Sexuality 69

Final Thought 76

THE END 81

CHAPTER ONE

INTRODUCTION

The need for an all-inclusive, thorough guide to sexual wellbeing is more than ever in a world where conversations about sexuality frequently stray into uncomfortable or forbidden areas. "Navigating Sexual Wellness" provides readers with a comprehensive approach to comprehending and improving their intimate lives, acting as a beacon of light in the frequently murky waters of sexual health.

Sexual wellbeing includes all facets of our lives physical, mental, emotional, and interpersonal and goes beyond the mere absence of illness.

This book aims to encourage readers to embrace their sexuality with authenticity and confidence by encouraging a deeper understanding of themselves and their relationships. It does this by doing more than merely solving problems.

You'll find a plethora of information covering a wide range of subjects in these pages, from intimacy-building activities to anatomy and physiology to the study of pleasure in all its manifestations. By utilizing empirical data and integrating viewpoints from psychology, sociology, and holistic medicine, this manual aims to give readers a road map for skillfully and compassionately navigating their sexual adventures.

The book "Navigating Sexual Wellness" is here to support you on your journey to happiness and fulfillment, whether your goals are to overcome obstacles, strengthen your relationship with your partner, or just broaden your awareness of human sexuality. It's an invitation to go on a path of self-discovery and development, embracing sexual wellness as a crucial component of our entire well-being. So let's set out on this journey together to achieve more holistic, vibrant, and gratifying approaches to sexual wellness and health.

The Basics of Sexual Health

The foundation of human well-being is sexual health, which has a significant impact on our emotional, mental, and physical conditions. However, navigating this element of our lives can be intimidating given the complexity of modern living. "Foundations of Sexual Health" offers a thorough examination of the essential ideas that guide a satisfying and all-encompassing approach to sexual health.

Sexual wellness is really much more than the absence of illness. It includes developing positive ideas on sexuality, having safe, consensual sexual encounters, and being able to have fulfilling, enjoyable intimate relationships. By giving readers a thorough understanding of these fundamental concepts, this book hopes to enable readers to set out on a path towards increased sexual fulfillment and self-discovery.

We shall delve into the complexities of sexual anatomy and physiology, solve the riddles of arousal and desire, and examine the psychological and emotional aspects of intimacy in these pages. Using knowledge from sociology, psychology, and public health, among other disciplines, we will explore how society shapes our ideas about sexuality and removes obstacles that frequently stand in the way of our ability to express it.

However, "Foundations of Sexual Health" is more than just a theoretical investigation; it is a useful manual created to give readers the skills and knowledge required to develop a meaningful and healthy sexual life. This book provides helpful guidance for negotiating the complexity of contemporary sexual relationships with confidence and integrity, covering everything from communication techniques and boundary-setting to contraception and STI prevention.

Let's acknowledge that, as we set out on this journey together, sexual health is a continuous process of self-awareness and personal development rather than a goal. We open the door to a more powerful, liberated, and satisfying understanding of sexuality by establishing these fundamental ideas one that recognizes the richness of human experience and the innate beauty of our common humanity.

Cultural and Historical Views of Sexuality

The Evolution of Sexual Norms and Beliefs in Ancient Civilizations

Sexuality was fundamental to ancient civilizations' rites, ideologies, and social structures during the earliest periods of human history. From the fertile banks of the Nile to the Mesopotamian valleys, religion, fertility ceremonies, and social customs were frequently entwined with sexuality.

The complex pantheon of gods and goddesses of ancient Egypt offers an intriguing prism through which to look at the relationship between spirituality and sexuality. In this culture, childbearing was vital to the success and survival of the society, and sexuality was regarded as a divine gift. The significance of reproduction and the life-and-death cycles were emphasized by the worship of fertility deities like Osiris and Isis.

Similar to this, the Gilgamesh epic in Mesopotamia provides insights into the views on sexuality that were common in Sumerian society at the time. In this society, sexuality was not just a personal issue but also a social one, and holy prostitutes acted as bridges between the spiritual and material worlds. It was thought that by performing these holy rituals, the community's welfare and the land's fertility would be guaranteed.

The ancient Greeks brought in an era of philosophical study and creative expression by migrating westward. In this instance, sexuality was examined with a breadth and nuance not found in antiquity. Greek society accepted a wide range of sexual expression, from the homoerotic partnerships revered in works like Plato's Symposium to the worship of Aphrodite, the goddess of beauty and love.

On the other hand, despite greatly appropriating Greek culture, the Roman Empire enforced more rigid moral standards and social stratification. Even though there is a lot of sexual imagery in Roman art and literature, women are still subjugated and gender roles are fixed. Although prostitution was quite popular, sexual behavior was strictly controlled, and adultery was illegal.

We start to notice themes and patterns emerging as we go through the history of ancient civilizations; these continue to influence how we currently interpret sexuality. The foundation for the intricate web of sexuality-related ideas and attitudes that would develop over millennia was set by ancient cultures, which integrated spirituality and sexuality and regulated sexual conduct through laws and social conventions.

Europe in the Middle Ages: Sexuality, Sin, and Redemption

During the Middle Ages, which were marked by intense religious fervor and social upheaval, Christianity solidified its position as the predominant moral and religious authority in Europe. Sexuality was progressively entwined with ideas of sin, morality, and redemption during this time, influencing attitudes and actions that would persist for centuries to come.

According to Christian doctrine, having sex is a necessary evil that should only be allowed in marriage and for the sake of having children. There was a strong emphasis on chastity and celibacy, especially among the clergy, and extramarital sex was viewed as a serious transgression. The Church imposed severe moral standards, punished sins with excommunication or even death, and exerted tremendous control over all facets of life, including sexual behavior.

But more sophisticated views of sexuality also emerged during the medieval era, coinciding with this widespread asceticism. Though it was limited to a socially acceptable framework, the idea of courtly love, made popular by troubadours and poets, emphasized the ideals of romantic love and sensual desire. The complex relationship between desire and morality in medieval Europe is reflected in this conflict between the romanticized ideas of love and the brutal realities of sexual repression.

Furthermore, since erotic literature, art, and folklore abound, the medieval era was defined by a fixation with the bizarre and the sensual. The tensions and contradictions inherent in medieval culture were reflected in the celebration and demonization of sexuality, which can be seen in everything from the cheeky stories found in Boccaccio's Decameron to the graphic iconography that adorned the walls of churches and castles.

We face the lingering effects of these contradictory views on sexuality when we dig farther into the medieval worldview. Our views of sex and morality in the modern world are still shaped by the residual effects of Christian morality as well as the relics of pagan fertility rites and folk customs. We can learn a great deal about the ongoing effort to balance the needs of the spirit with the wants of the flesh by delving into the complexity of sexuality in medieval Europe.

A profound change in Western thought was ushered in by the Renaissance and Enlightenment, which brought with them humanism, science, and the rediscovering of classical knowledge. New perspectives on the body, the self, and human relationships were made possible by a significant shift in attitudes regarding sexuality against the backdrop of increased intellectual freedom and cultural prosperity.

The Renaissance saw a resurgence of interest in the human body and its pleasures due to the revival of classical art and literature. While writers like Petrarch and Boccaccio tackled themes of love, desire, and sexuality in their works, artists like Michelangelo and Leonardo da Vinci embraced the beauty and sensuality of the human body. This celebration of sensuality and the body marked a shift away from the asceticism of the Middle Ages and toward a more accepting and free sexuality.

The Enlightenment pushed for reason, individuality, and personal liberty, further challenging conventional ideas of morality and authority. Philosophers like Voltaire and John Locke defended people's freedom to pursue their own happiness and fulfillment without being restricted by social norms or religious doctrine. Modern ideas of sexual freedom and personal autonomy were shaped by this emphasis on reason and human agency.

In addition, new scientific theories and medical discoveries of the Enlightenment completely changed our perception of human sexuality. Pioneers in anatomy and physiology, like Andreas Vesalius and William Harvey, illuminated the intricacies of arousal and desire as well as the workings of sexual reproduction. These scientific breakthroughs disproved moral taboos and prevalent myths, opening the door for a more enlightened and knowledgeable understanding of sexuality.

The Enlightenment was not without its paradoxes and limitations, nevertheless, despite these advancements.

CHAPTER TWO

Deeply ingrained societal hierarchies and inequities, notably with regard to gender and sexuality, coexisted with the exaltation of reason and independence. With patriarchal norms and expectations limiting their sexual agency, women in particular continued to be marginalized and subjugated.

We face the continuing contradictions between freedom and confinement, reason and superstition, which continue to define our view of sexuality today, as we consider the legacies of the Renaissance and Enlightenment. Examining the intellectual and cultural currents of these revolutionary times helps us understand how human sexuality is changing and how the pursuit of freedom, equality, and self-expression has persisted throughout history.

Victorian Ethics and the Development of Sexuality

The libertarian attitude of the Renaissance and Enlightenment stands in stark contrast to the strict moral norms and social conservatism of the Victorian era. During this time, sexuality was seen more and more through the prism of morality and social order, with stringent regulations dictating acceptable sexual behavior.

In Victorian society, morality and respectability were highly valued, especially when it came to issues of gender and sexuality. The ideals of piety, purity, and domesticity were elevated by the cult of domesticity, which also elevated women's status as moral stewards of the home and family. A rigorous sexual hierarchy was established as a result of the widespread belief in the value of childbearing and the sanctity of marriage, with men and women expected to fulfill their assigned tasks.

Physiology and Anatomy of the Biological Basis of Sex

A complex interaction of biological, psychological, and social elements determines human sexuality. The complex anatomy and physiology that controls our sensations of arousal, reproduction, and desire is at the center of it all. Comprehending the biological underpinnings of sexuality is essential to appreciating the subtleties of human sexuality and advancing sexual health and welfare. This chapter explores the structures and mechanisms that underlie our sexual experiences as we dig into the anatomy and physiology of sex.

Structure of Sexual Organs:

The core of human sexuality is found in the reproductive organs, which produce gametes (eggs in females, sperm in males) and facilitate sexual activity. The testes, which generate sperm and secrete testosterone, the hormone in charge of secondary sexual characteristic development, are one of the principal sex organs in males. During sexual contact, sperm are delivered through the penis, which is made of erectile tissue.

The ovaries, which generate eggs and exude the hormones progesterone and estrogen which are crucial for controlling the menstrual cycle and promoting pregnancy are the main sex organs in females. The female reproductive tract is made up of the vagina, cervix, and uterus, which aid in sperm transfer, fertilization, and gestation.

Males and females differ from one another in secondary sexual traits that extend beyond the primary sex organs and influence mate choice and sexual attraction. These traits are more prevalent in men and include growing facial and body hair, a deeper voice, and larger muscles. Secondary sexual traits in females include the development of breasts, wider hips, and body fat distribution.

The Physiology of the Sexual Reaction

The range of physiological alterations that take place during sexual engagement is included in the sexual response cycle. Four stages usually make up the phase:

Resolve, orgasm, plateau, and excitement

People have increased blood flow to their genital organs during the excitation phase, which causes erectile tissue to engorge and the vaginal walls to lubricate. In anticipation of sexual activity, there is an increase in heart rate, blood pressure, and muscle tension.

The excitement phase's physiological alterations are maintained during the plateau phase, which is characterized by increased vaginal blood flow and muscle tension. Males develop a completely extended penis, while females experience heightened sensitivity and desire because to blood swells in the clitoris and labia.

The pelvic muscles flex rhythmically during the orgasmic phase, releasing sexual tension and producing powerful feelings of release and pleasure. An orgasm in a male is usually accompanied by ejaculation, whereas in a female, pelvic muscular contractions and a subjective feeling of release are indicative.

The last stage of the resolution phase is the gradual restoration of normal physiological functioning after an orgasm. Heart rate and blood pressure return to normal, genital vasocongestion lessens, and muscle tension eases.

Gaining knowledge about the biological underpinnings of sex can help us better understand the systems regulating our sexual experiences. Understanding the complex anatomy and physiology involved can help people have a better understanding of their bodies and sexual reactions, which can lead to the development of positive attitudes toward sexuality and the promotion of sexual well-being. We shall examine how these biological elements combine with psychological and social aspects to shape human sexuality as a whole in the upcoming chapters.

Gender Identity and Sexual Orientation

Gender identity and sexual orientation are essential components of human variation, involving the intricate interactions between biological, psychological, and social elements that influence people's perceptions of identity, attraction, and self-expression. Promoting inclusivity, upholding individual autonomy, and cultivating a more just and affirming society all depend on having a solid understanding of sexual orientation and gender identity. This chapter delves into the subtleties of gender identity and sexual orientation, examining the various ways that people feel and express their gender and sexuality.

Orientation towards Sexuality:

A person's pattern of emotional, romantic, and sexual attraction to other people is referred to as their sexual orientation. Sexual orientation is a spectrum that encompasses a wide range of identities and experiences, despite being commonly classified as heterosexual (attraction to individuals of the opposite gender), homosexual (attraction to individuals of the same gender), or bisexual (attraction to individuals of multiple genders).

While some people's sexual orientation is variable and changes over time, for others it is set and remains constant throughout their life. Although there are a number of factors that may influence sexual orientation, including hormones, genetics, and early experiences, it is ultimately a very personal element of identity that cannot be explained by straightforward biology or environmental factors.

Identity of Gender:

An individual's internal sense of gender, which may or may not correspond with the sex given to them at birth, is referred to as gender identity. Many people identify as cisgender, which is the gender they were assigned at birth. However, some people identify as transgender, which is a different gender, or as non-binary, genderqueer, genderfluid, or anywhere else outside the standard binary of male and female.

Biological sex, which refers to the anatomical and physiological traits connected to being male or female, is not the same as gender identity. Gender identity is deeply established and can be changed by a combination of biological, psychological, and social variables, whereas sex is normally assigned at birth based on anatomical traits.

Getting Around Diversity:

The variety of sexual orientations and gender identities that exist within society must be acknowledged and respected. Based on sexual orientation or gender identity, discrimination, stigma, and marginalization can have a significant negative impact on people's wellbeing and increase the risk of violence, social exclusion, and mental health inequalities.

Promoting everyone's health and wellbeing, regardless of sexual orientation or gender identity, requires the creation of inclusive cultures that value and celebrate variety. This entails giving people access to affirming healthcare, anti-discrimination laws, and all-encompassing education that recognizes the range of human variation.

Gender identity and sexual orientation are intricate and multidimensional facets of human identity that are difficult to classify into neat categories. Through acknowledging the multiplicity of experiences and manifestations within the LGBTQ+ community, we can establish a fairer and more comprehensive community that honors and reveres the innate dignity and value of each person, irrespective of their gender identity or sexual orientation. In the chapters that follow, we'll delve into the distinct struggles and experiences that people on the LGBTQ+ spectrum encounter and talk about tactics for fostering empowerment, acceptance, and understanding.

Encouraging the Health of Sexuality

The physical, emotional, and social facets of sexuality are all part of sexual health, which is an essential element of general wellbeing.

Encouraging positive attitudes toward sexuality, offering reliable information and tools, and establishing settings that encourage healthy sexual relationships and behaviors are all part of promoting sexual health. We look at methods in this chapter that can be used to promote sexual health on an individual, interpersonal, and social level.

Understanding and Awareness:

Encouraging sexual health requires comprehensive sexual education because it gives people the information and tools they need to make wise choices about their relationships and sexual well-being. A wide range of subjects are covered in effective sexual education programs, such as anatomy and physiology, consent and communication techniques, STI prevention and contraception, and the value of healthy relationships and limits.

Sexual health promotion also requires destigmatizing discussions about sexuality and raising awareness of it. We may enable people to look for information, ask questions, and speak up for their own sexual health needs by dispelling myths and misconceptions about sex and sexuality and establishing accepting, conversational environments.

Healthcare Accessibility:

Encouraging sexual health and well-being requires having access to comprehensive and affirming healthcare services. Healthcare professionals ought to receive culturally competent, inclusive treatment that takes into account each patient's particular needs and experiences, regardless of their sexual orientation or gender identity.

Encouraging people to take charge of their sexual health and make educated decisions about their bodies and relationships requires guaranteeing access to a comprehensive range of sexual and reproductive health services, such as contraception, STI testing and treatment, and sexual health counseling.

Conducive Conditions:

Promoting sexual health and lowering stigma and discrimination need the establishment of welcoming cultures that celebrate and affirm diversity. Policies and practices that support inclusivity, respect people's autonomy and agency, and remove structural obstacles to sexual health and well-being should be implemented in workplaces, schools, and communities.

Establishing wholesome and constructive connections, whether platonic or intimate, is another aspect of supportive surroundings. In partnerships, encouraging consent, open communication, and respect for one another can help avoid sexual assault, foster emotional closeness, and improve general wellbeing.

Campaigning for Social Change:

Promoting sexual health at the societal level can be effectively accomplished through advocacy and social change. Advocating for comprehensive sexual education, opposing discrimination based on sexual orientation, gender identity, or other variables, and opposing laws and policies that compromise sexual health and rights are all important tasks for advocates and activists.

We can build a more just and equitable society where everyone has the chance to attain optimal sexual health and well-being by increasing knowledge, energizing communities, and pushing for structural change.

A multimodal strategy that takes into account societal, interpersonal, and individual aspects is needed to promote sexual health. We can create a society free from stigma, prejudice, and violence where everyone has the opportunity to enjoy healthy and full sexual lives by placing a high priority on education, access to healthcare, supportive surroundings, and activism for social change. We will look at particular tactics and programs for enhancing sexual health and wellbeing in a variety of contexts and demographics in the upcoming chapters.

Taking Care of Sexual Disorders and Dysfunction

A person's physical, emotional, and social well-being can all be adversely affected by sexual dysfunction and disorders, which can have a substantial negative influence on their quality of life. It is necessary to address sexual dysfunction and disorders by having access to supportive interventions and effective treatments, as well as by having a thorough awareness of the underlying causes and contributing variables. This chapter examines the many forms of sexual dysfunction and disorders, their causes, and methods for diagnosis, counseling, and support.

Sexual dysfunction and disorders: categories

A wide range of issues with sexual arousal, desire, orgasm, and pain are included in sexual dysfunction. Several common forms of sexual dysfunction include low libido (reduced desire for sexual activity), delayed ejaculation (difficulty ejaculating), premature ejaculation (difficulty achieving or maintaining an erection), and sexual pain disorders (such as dyspareunia and vaginismus).

Contrarily, sexual disorders are characterized by recurring sexual behavior patterns that are upsetting or interfere with functioning. Sexual aversion disorder (strong dislike to sexual activity), paraphilic disorders (persistent sexual arousal to unusual items, settings, or thoughts), and hypoactive sexual desire disorder (consistently low or absent sexual desire) are a few examples of sexual illnesses.

Sexual Dysfunction and Disorders Causes:

Physical, psychological, and relationship variables are just a few of the underlying reasons of sexual dysfunction and diseases. Sexually dysfunctional drugs (e.g., antidepressants, antihypertensives) and medical diseases including diabetes, heart disease, and hormone imbalances can also lead to problems with reproduction.

The emergence or worsening of sexual dysfunction and disorders can also be significantly influenced by psychological factors such as stress, anxiety, depression, and traumatic experiences in the past. Problems with relationships, communication, and cultural or religious views on sex may all be contributing factors to challenges with sexual functioning.

Evaluation and Intervention:

An extensive assessment of a patient's medical history, psychological variables, interpersonal dynamics, and sexual practices is usually required for the diagnosis of sexual dysfunction and disorders. To evaluate sexual functioning and find any underlying problems, medical professionals may employ laboratory testing, physical examinations, and standardized questionnaires.

Depending on the precise diagnosis and underlying causes, there are many approaches to treating sexual dysfunction and diseases.

CHAPTER THREE

Medication (such as phosphodiesterase inhibitors for erectile dysfunction, hormone therapy for hormonal imbalances) and surgical procedures (such as penile implants for severe erectile dysfunction) are examples of medical therapies.

Psychological therapies that target the underlying psychological causes of sexual dysfunction include mindfulness-based therapies, cognitive-behavioral therapy (CBT), and sex therapy. Enhancing communication and closeness, as well as addressing relationship problems, are possible benefits of couples therapy.

Interventions that Provide Support:

When it comes to treating sexual dysfunction and disorders, supportive interventions can be just as important as medical and psychological treatments. Peer therapy, online forums, and support groups can provide people a sense of belonging and validation, which helps lessen the shame and loneliness that come with having sexual troubles.

In order to help people and their partners understand the nature of sexual dysfunction and disorders, lessen anxiety and stigma, and improve coping mechanisms and communication skills, education and psychoeducation are also crucial parts of supportive therapies.

A multidisciplinary approach that recognises the intricate interplay of biological, psychological, and relational components is necessary to address sexual dysfunction and disorders. Healthcare professionals have the ability to assist people and their partners in overcoming sexual challenges and improving their general well-being and contentment with their sexual lives by offering thorough assessments, efficient treatment options, and supportive interventions. We shall examine particular strategies and treatments for treating sexual dysfunction and disorders in various populations and situations in the ensuing chapters.

Increasing Satisfaction and Sexual Pleasure

Physical pleasure, emotional closeness, and general life satisfaction are all influenced by sexual pleasure and satisfaction, which are essential elements of human well-being. A deeper understanding of one's own preferences and needs, the development of good communication skills, and the exploration of methods and practices that foster intimacy and pleasure are all necessary for improving sexual enjoyment and fulfillment. This chapter looks at methods for improving sex satisfaction and pleasure on an individual basis as well as in close partnerships.

Comprehending Eroticism:

A wide range of physiological events, psychological states, and emotional sensations that support emotions of arousal, fullness, and satisfaction are together referred to as sexual pleasure. The key to optimizing pleasure and happiness is having a thorough understanding of one's own sexual responses and preferences.

Investigating and Testing:

Individuals and couples can learn what makes them happy and satisfied by experimenting with various sexual expression, methods, and pursuits. This could include playing with sexy dreams, experimenting with different positions, including sex toys or accessories, or investigating sensual touch and massage.

Honest Communication

Enhancing sexual pleasure and happiness in close relationships requires effective communication. This entails being transparent and honest about your preferences, boundaries, and desires; paying attention to and honoring your partner's needs and aspirations; and offering constructive criticism and support when engaging in sexual activity.

Developing Close Emotional Bonds:

Satisfying sexual relationships are built on emotional closeness, which encourages vulnerability, trust, and connection between lovers. Prioritizing quality time spent together, fostering mutual respect and understanding, and expressing love and affection both within and outside of the bedroom are all important components of developing emotional intimacy.

Being Present and Mindful:

Through complete immersion in the moment and connection with their sensations and emotions, practicing mindfulness and presence during sexual relations can increase pleasure and fulfillment. In order to engage in mindful sex, one must pay attention to the present, tune into their body's feelings, and develop an awareness of both their own and their partner's reactions.

Investigating Sensuality

A wide variety of sensory experiences that support and enhance sexual fulfillment are included in the concept of sensuality. This could involve investigating sensory-enhancing techniques like sexual massage or sensory deprivation, as well as indulging in sensual activities like kissing, snuggling, or taking a bath together.

Taking Care of Sexual Issues:

Sustaining sexual pleasure and happiness over time requires addressing potential issues or problems. This could entail resolving interpersonal problems that might be affecting one's sexual health, looking into medical therapies for sexual dysfunction, or getting professional assistance from a sex therapist or counselor.

Improving one's sexual enjoyment and fulfillment is a continuous process that calls for curiosity, openness, and a readiness to learn about and interact with oneself and one's partner. Individuals and couples can enjoy more fulfillment and happiness in their sexual lives by exploring strategies and practices that encourage pleasure and closeness, establishing effective communication skills, and having a deeper understanding of their own desires and preferences. We will look at particular methods and strategies for improving sexual satisfaction and pleasure in a variety of settings and demographics in the upcoming chapters.

Healthy Sexual Behavior Throughout Life

A person's sexual health is a dynamic and complex part of their overall well-being that changes throughout their lifetime. People go through changes in their bodies, relationships, and sexual desires and behaviors from birth to old age. Acknowledging the distinct requirements and obstacles encountered by individuals at varying phases of life is crucial for comprehending and advocating for sexual health throughout life. This chapter examines the many facets of sexual health from early childhood to old age and talks about methods for fostering contentment and well-being at each point.

Early Life and Childhood:

Early childhood is a critical period for sexual health as people learn about relationships, permission, limits, and body awareness. In order to promote a good and accepting attitude toward sexuality throughout this stage, caregivers must provide age-appropriate knowledge, set an example of healthy relationships, and create spaces that encourage self-exploration and discovery.

Teenage years:

Puberty begins and sexual identity and relationships are explored during adolescence, a time of fast physical, emotional, and social development. Adolescent sexual health promotion include giving young people access to accurate and thorough sexual education, addressing their questions and concerns in an open, nonjudgmental manner, and enabling them to make decisions about their bodies and relationships.

Early Adulthood:

In terms of sexuality, young adulthood is a time for experimentation, self-discovery, and exploration. People can explore their sexual wants and preferences, negotiate their first sexual experiences, and form meaningful relationships. Encouraging open communication, engaging in safer sexual activities, and cultivating a positive body image and self-confidence are all important aspects of promoting sexual health in young adults.

Growing Up:

The experiences and phases of life that make up adulthood are diverse and include everything from establishing a family and raising children to pursuing professional objectives and sustaining close connections. In order to promote sexual health into maturity, it is important to address the particular difficulties and pressures that individuals and couples encounter, such as managing stress, striking a balance between work and family obligations, and adjusting to changes in sexual desire and satisfaction.

Midlife:

Changes in relationships, identity, and physical health are hallmarks of midlife, a time of introspection and transition. This may require adjusting to shifts in sexual desire, function, or satisfaction for some people, or it may be a period of sexual reawakening and exploration for others. Encouraging closeness and connection in relationships, addressing age-related changes in sexual functioning, and assisting people in maintaining a pleasant and meaningful sexual life are all part of promoting sexual health during midlife.

Advanced Age:

When it comes to sexual health, becoming older has its own advantages and disadvantages. Older adults can still enjoy intimacy, pleasure, and connection through sexual activity and intimacy, even when physical changes and health issues may affect sexual function and desire. Encouraging older adults' sexual health entails addressing age-related issues and medical conditions, giving them access to resources and services that support them, and creating a culture that values and respects their sexual agency and overall well-being.

A lifetime adventure, sexual health changes and evolves with time. We may encourage a more inclusive and affirming approach to sexual health that acknowledges and respects the range of human experiences and wants by acknowledging the particular needs and difficulties faced by people at different stages of life. We shall look at certain tactics and programs for enhancing sexual health and wellbeing across the life course in the upcoming chapters.

Social and Cultural Aspects of Sexual Health

In addition to personal experiences and actions, cultural and community conventions, values, and attitudes toward sexuality have a significant impact on sexual health. Beliefs regarding sex, gender roles, sexual habits, and access to resources and services related to sexual health are greatly influenced by cultural and societal variables. This chapter examines the ways that society and cultural factors affect sexual health outcomes and offers tactics for advancing a more affirming, equitable, and inclusive approach to sexual health in a variety of cultural contexts.

Cultural Principles and Beliefs:

Many nations and cultural groups have quite varied cultural views and values regarding sexuality. These ideas may have an impact on perceptions of gender roles, marriage, sexual expression, and family dynamics. For instance, societies that place a high importance on family honor and collectivism might be more concerned with maintaining conventional gender roles and keeping virginity until marriage, whereas cultures that value individualism and autonomy might be more interested in promoting gender equality and sexual freedom.

Moral and Religious Viewpoints:

Moral and religious convictions frequently have a big impact on how people feel about sexuality and sexual activity. The teachings of various faith traditions on topics like abortion, contraception, premarital sex, and LGBTQ+ rights might affect people's access to resources and knowledge on sexual health. Regarding specific sexual activities or identities, stigma, prejudice, and shame may also be influenced by religious and moral viewpoints.

Social Expectations and Norms:

People's actions and decisions about relationships, sex, and reproductive health are influenced by social norms and expectations surrounding sexuality. These norms may specify what constitutes appropriate sexual expression, establish gender roles and expectations, and have an impact on choices on when and with whom to have sex. People who violate sexual standards may face discrimination, social exclusion, and stigma, which may cause them to repress or hide their sexual identities and urges.

Obtaining Resources for Sexual Health:

The resources and services available to those seeking sexual health can be greatly impacted by societal factors, including but not limited to socioeconomic background, race, ethnicity, gender identity, and sexual orientation. Disparities in sexual health outcomes can be made worse by structural injustices and systemic obstacles, such as discrimination in healthcare settings, a lack of comprehensive sexual education, restricted access to STI testing and contraception, and prejudice in the medical community.

Cultural Sensitivity in Genital Health:

It takes a culturally competent approach that respects and accepts the values, beliefs, and practices of many cultural groups to promote sexual health in diverse cultural situations. Healthcare professionals and educators need to be aware of cultural variances, confront taboos related to sexuality in both culture and religion, and customize sexual health programs to the particular requirements and preferences of various communities.

Attitudes toward sexuality, availability of tools for sexual health, and health results are significantly shaped by cultural and societal factors. We may create more successful methods for promoting sexual well-being that are inclusive, respectful, and sensitive to the varied needs and experiences of individuals and communities if we acknowledge the intricate interaction of cultural influences in influencing sexual health. We will examine particular interventions and strategies for enhancing sexual health in various cultural contexts and groups in the ensuing chapters.

In order to improve sexual health and well-being, it is imperative that people have access to trustworthy information, support networks, and medical professionals. It can be intimidating to navigate the wide range of information accessible, though. We identify a number of resources in this chapter that people can use to get reliable information, assistance, and services regarding sexual health.

Education on Sexual Health:

Accurate knowledge about anatomy, contraception, STI prevention, consent, and healthy relationships is made available to people through comprehensive sexual health education programs. On a variety of sexual health-related topics, reliable sources like textbooks, websites, and instructional materials from groups like Planned Parenthood, the American Sexual Health Association, and the World Health Organization provide insightful information.

Providers of Healthcare:

In order to promote sexual health and resolve issues, healthcare professionals such as urologists, gynecologists, primary care physicians, and sexual health specialists are essential. People can look for medical professionals who understand sexual health issues, offer nonjudgmental care, and provide services including STI testing, contraception counseling, and therapy for sexual dysfunction.

Clinics for Sexual Health:

Specialized services pertaining to sexual and reproductive health are provided by sexual health clinics. These clinics may offer sexual health education, pregnancy testing and choices counseling, STI testing and treatment, and contraception advice and services. Numerous sexual health clinics promote confidentiality and nonjudgmental care while providing low-cost or free services.

Therapy & Counseling:

For those with relationship problems, mental pain related to sexuality, or sexual worries, counseling and therapy can be very helpful. Individual or couples counseling is available from licensed psychologists, therapists, and sex workers to treat a variety of sexual health difficulties, such as gender identity exploration, intimacy challenges, and sexual dysfunction.

Helplines and Hotlines:

Hotlines and helplines provide people in need with private support and information.

CHAPTER FOUR

Resource and support for victims of sexual assault, victims of relationship abuse, and LGBTQ+ people in distress are offered by organizations including the Trevor Project, the National Sexual Assault Hotline, and the National Domestic Violence Hotline.

Online forums and communities:

Online forums and groups can offer a helpful setting where people can interact with one another, exchange stories, and get resources and information about sexual health. Peer support, professional guidance, and educational resources on a variety of sexual health problems are available on websites and forums including

Scarleteen, the r/sex community on Reddit, and the sexual health area of Healthline.

Advocacy and Assistance Groups:

Advocacy and support groups employ education, advocacy, and direct services to advance sexual health, rights, and justice. Resources, support, and advocacy for sexual health and rights are offered by groups including the Guttmacher Institute, the Sexuality Information and Education Council of the United States (SIECUS), and neighborhood LGBTQ+ community centers.

In order to improve sexual health and well-being, it is imperative that people have access to trustworthy information, support networks, and medical professionals. People can access the information and support they need to make informed decisions about their sexual health and lead fulfilling and healthy lives by making use of resources like advocacy and support organizations, healthcare providers, sexual health clinics, hotlines and helplines, counseling and therapy services, online communities and forums, and sexual health education programs. We'll look at some specific methods for getting to and using these resources in the upcoming chapters.

Accepting Liberation and Authenticity in Sexuality

To be truly honest and liberated from shame and criticism over one's sexuality, one must embrace their true identities, wants, and expressions. In a world where sexuality is frequently associated with taboos, conventions, and expectations from society, embracing authenticity and emancipation can be a life-changing path towards fulfillment, empowerment, and self-discovery. This chapter delves into the significance of accepting sexual authenticity and emancipation, as well as methods for regaining control, enjoyment, and delight in one's sexual encounters.

Comprehending the Concept of Sexual Authenticity:

Respecting and expressing one's actual limits, identities, and desires in accordance with one's values and beliefs is a necessary component of being authentically sexual. It necessitates accepting all facets of one's sexuality, fantasies, orientations, preferences, and desires without worrying about being rejected or judged. Accepting one's sexual agency and autonomy and declining to fit in with social standards or expectations that don't reflect one's actual self are key components of embracing sexual authenticity.

Defying Social Expectations and Norms:

Shame, stigma, and discrimination are frequently sustained by societal norms and expectations surrounding sexuality, especially with regard to marginalized communities and non-normative sexualities. Defying these expectations and promoting a more accepting and encouraging view of sexuality are necessary steps toward embracing sexual authenticity and liberty. This could entail fighting against heteronormativity, questioning gender norms, and promoting justice and sexual rights for all people.

Regaining Happiness and Pleasure:

Regaining pleasure and delight may be a profound act of self-love and emancipation in a culture that frequently places a premium on performance, perfection, and achievement in sexuality. Prioritizing pleasure, curiosity, and connection over conforming to outside norms or expectations is a key component of embracing sexual authenticity. This might entail developing a healthy relationship with one's body and sexuality as well as investigating novel feelings, fantasies, or fulfilling pursuits.

Examining Expression and Identity:

A great variety of identities, orientations, and manifestations are included in sexual authenticity, and each one is worthy of acceptance, dignity, and affirmation. Exploring and embracing one's own identity and expression—whether it conforms to or defies social norms is a crucial part of embracing sexual authenticity. This could entail supporting various gender and sexual expressions, accepting non-binary or fluid identities, or coming out as LGBTQ+.

Fostering Respect and Consent:

The development of consent, respect, and moral behavior in sexual interactions is essential to sexual authenticity and liberty. Prioritizing consent and communication, honoring limits and needs, and promoting satisfaction and fulfillment for both parties are all part of embracing sexual authenticity. Investigating ethical non-monogamy, giving enthusiastic permission, and dispelling myths about entitlement or compulsion in sexual encounters are some ways to achieve this.

Honoring Intersectionality and Diversity:

Recognizing the interdependence of sexuality with other facets of identity, such as race, ethnicity, class, ability, and religion, sexual authenticity and emancipation are intrinsically intersectional. Advocating for social justice and equity in sexual health and rights, as well as valuing the diversity of human experiences and manifestations, are all part of embracing sexual authenticity.

Accepting one's sexual emancipation and authenticity is a profoundly personal and life-changing path to fulfillment, empowerment, and self-discovery. People can regain control over their sexuality and lead more genuine, contented, and free lives by questioning society norms and expectations, reclaiming joy and pleasure, investigating identity and expression, developing consent and respect, and celebrating diversity and intersectionality. We will look at certain tactics and approaches for embracing sexual emancipation and authenticity in various settings and cultures in the upcoming chapters.

Final Thought

It's important to consider the powerful path that lies ahead as we get to the end of our investigation into sexual wellbeing. Your sexual well-being is an ongoing journey of empowerment, self-improvement, and self-discovery rather than a destination. You may manage your sexual journey with confidence, honesty, and joy by adhering to the principles of sexual health, developing self-awareness, and speaking up for your needs and desires.

We've covered a wide range of topics related to sexual wellbeing in this book, including the biological underpinnings of sex, societal influences, encouraging self-care, and embracing authenticity and liberation. We've talked about how to improve your sexual well-being at any stage of life and in a variety of cultural situations, as well as how to handle problems and find resources.

Self-awareness and self-compassion are the first steps towards empowering your sexual journey. Investigate your preferences, boundaries, and desires for a while without guilt or condemnation. Pay attention to your body, respect your wants, and put your enjoyment and contentment first. Keep in mind that sexual wellbeing includes emotional intimacy, relational fulfillment, and the development of meaningful connections in addition to physical health.

Speaking up for your rights and sexual health is another essential component of empowerment. Speak up in favor of inclusive policies that support everyone's right to sexual health, regardless of gender, identity, or orientation, as well as for comprehensive sexual education and healthcare access. Push for a culture that values diversity, consent, and respect by challenging cultural norms and expectations that support sexuality-related stigma, discrimination, and shame.

Finally, keep in mind that you are unique in your sexual adventure. Celebrate the complexity and diversity of human sexuality, embrace your honesty, and investigate your impulses. Look for professionals, resources, and groups that will encourage and assist you on your journey. Embrace your sexual adventure with curiosity and confidence. It may be a source of fulfillment, pleasure, and empowerment.

May every step of your road towards sexual empowerment bring you happiness, contentment, and freedom. It is essential to your identity to embrace, respect, and celebrate your sexuality. With the right information, self-awareness, and empowerment, you can design a sexual life that is genuine, satisfying, and entirely your own.

Cheers to accepting your sexual journey with bravery, empathy, and self-determination. I hope the trip is one of joy, progress, and discovery.

THE END